DAPOXETINE USAGE GUIDE

A comprehensive guidebook on all you need to know about Dapoxetine to cure erectile dysfunction

Dr. Nathan Andrews

Contents

CHAPTER ONE

Introduction to Dapoxetine

Dapoxetine is an antidepressant drug mainly indicated for the treatment of PE in male patients. It comes under a group of drugs called selective serotonin reuptake inhibitors (SSRI) which are majorly prescribed in

Contents

CHAPTER ONE

Introduction to Dapoxetine

Dapoxetine is an antidepressant drug mainly indicated for the treatment of PE in male patients. It comes under a group of drugs called selective serotonin reuptake inhibitors (SSRI) which are majorly prescribed in depressants and anxiety. However, dapoxetine is a part of the SSRI family drugs with a difference, which are developed to be taken on an as-needed basis and not daily and are therefore effective for the treatment of PE.

History and Development

The research of dapoxetine was launched in the early of the year 2000. First, it was explored with regard to its effect on depression since it is an SSRI. But the facts were revealed in clinical trials, it has a quick response time and a short span of effect which was not suitable for the patient with depression but for the ones who suffered from premature ejaculation. Further research was conducted on this chemical treatment and consequently its development shifted and it was formulated as well as tested for the treatment of PE.

Several countries' approving authorities have approved dapoxetine from 2008 starting with Finland, followed by other European countries, Asia and several Middle East countries. It has trade names in the market such as Priligy among others across the world.

Mechanism of Action

Dapoxetine under the category of selective serotonin reuptake inhibitor decreases the reuptake of serotonin into presynaptic neurons. This inhibition increases the amount of serotonin in the synaptic cleft and promotes neurotransmission while also delaying the time to ejaculation. Though the processes and interactions of serotonin ejaculation have not been fully described, what is known is that it is related to the activity in the central nervous system with respect to sexual function.

Derived from the above characteristics, dapoxetine

Mechanism of Action

Dapoxetine under the category of selective serotonin reuptake inhibitor decreases the reuptake of serotonin into presynaptic neurons. This inhibition increases the amount of serotonin in the synaptic cleft and promotes neurotransmission while also delaying the time to ejaculation. Though the processes and interactions of serotonin ejaculation have not been fully described, what is known is that it is related to the activity in the central nervous system with respect to sexual function.

Derived from the above characteristics, dapoxetine

has fast absorption and elimination rates hence can be used on demand. The substance can be used about one to three hours before sexual activity and once ingested, it can greatly assist in delaying ejaculation for some time thus affording a man better control over his ejaculatory process thus reducing on the symptoms of premature ejaculation.

Duration of Effect

The primary effective window is usually 1 to 3 hours after administering the substance commonly referred to as dapoxetine. Regarding the changes that occur in men's bodies during this period, the maximum positive effect can be noted in terms of postponed ejaculation.

The maximum results can be noticed within the first hours of the treatment, but some men may notice the positive outcomes up to 4 to 6 hours after the administration of the treatment, although the intensity may be weaker.

At times despite the effectiveness of the drug, several side effects may occur:

Dapoxetine is an SSRI with a special focus on the treatment of PE; like any other drug, dapoxetine has mild to severe side effects.

The mild side effects include dizziness, headaches, nightmares, loose stools, and nausea, abdominal pain and other PMS related side effects, anxiety, and mood swings.

Measures to be Taken While Undergoing the Process of Dapoxetine Intake

The consumption of dapoxetine in patients diagnosed with premature ejaculation requires several precautions to guarantee therapy efficacy as well as to reduce the possibility of side effects or adverse reactions. Here are key precautions to consider:Here are key precautions to consider:

1. One must take dapoxetine in the way that has been recommended by a qualified healthcare professional.

Incorrect dosages of a medicine may prove perilous as they cause side effects or decrease efficacy of the medicine. Besides, it is essential to avoid taking several tablets in a single day, within a 24-hour duration. Begin with the quantity that is prescribed which is normally 30 mg and only double it to 60 mg when prescribed.

2. Remember to look for symptoms as reactions like rash, itching, swelling, severe dizziness, trouble breathing. Since allergic reactions may sometimes be severe and warrant a trip to the hospitals, people who have the same should ensure

that they have a suitable and reliable identity management solution. . Consult a doctor if you experience any side effect that may be as a result of an allergy or any other reaction.

3. Do not drink alcohol while being on dapoxetine treatment. As alcohol can

increase the dangers of side effects of Dapoxetine such as dizziness, sleeping disorders, and poor decision-making abilities.

Also, it is recommended that one cuts on the consumption of alcohol during the period of treatment to avoid any complications. Use of other medications that should be combined with a certain measure of caution includes, other SSRI's MAO's, thioridazine, and some pain medicines.

4. Another side effect that may be attributed to dapoxetine is dizziness and also drowsiness. Such side effects will make it difficult for you to carry out tasks that

need clear understanding and coordination.

Therefore, it will be advisable not to drive or use machinery that is weighty in any way until you are alert to how dapoxetine has on you.

CHAPTER TWO

Negative Interactions of Dapoxetine

As much as dapoxetine is an effective drug to treat erectile dysfunctions, it has been noted to have a negative interaction with some drugs, certain substances and some medical conditions.

Thus, the intake of dapoxetine jointly with other medicines that influence serotonin levels, such as selective serotonin reuptake inhibitors (SSRIs) and serotonin-norepinephrine reuptake inhibitors (SNRIs), may result in serotonin syndrome, a severe condition due to excessive amounts of serotonin in the brain. Thus, they should not be used together, and one should report the administration of such medications to their healthcare provider.

Describes that Drugs from the class of MONOAMINE OXIDASE INHIBITORS can also affect serotonin levels increasing them and when combined with dapoxetine they can result in serotonin syndrome. In this regard, it is advisable to avoid the concurrent use of dapoxetine and MAOI; the use of either of the two should be at least 14 days after termination of the other. Some drugs raise the levels of dapoxetine in the blood due to the inhibition of metabolism, which can prove to be dangerous: Ketoconazole, itraconazole, ritonavir, and some antibiotics including clarithromycin. Therefore, it is recommended to notify your doctor if you are using any potent CYP3A4 inhibitors as the dosage of your medicine may need to be changed.

Thus, certain medication, substance use and activities should be avoided to get the best benefit of dapoxetine and to prevent unwanted side effects. Ensure that you reveal all your medical history, the kind of drugs and supplements that you are taking, and any underlying health conditions you have before taking dapoxetine. This will ensure that all possible interactions are effectively managed and the overall treatment plan is most effectively improved.

Common Side Effects

Regardless of the effectiveness of this

medication. It can also cause mild and temporary side effects such as headaches, abdominal pain, anxiety, nausea, diarrhea, and several others. Consult a medical doctor if you experience these side effects, as well as the severely damaging reactions that may occur.

Serious Prolonged Consequence of Dapoxetine

Like every other drug, it comes with severe long-term complications; these are mainly complicated by improper use of the drug or where certain allied factors exist. Information about such possibilities is beneficial in its utilization and the identification of any undesirable consequences.

Thus, long-term use of dapoxetine enhances the probability of worsening of initial heart diseases or the occurrence of new ones. Thus, constant control of the cardiovascular system is critical, particularly in cases of existing cardiovascular diseases. Any alteration or development of new symptoms related to cardiovascular diseases should be presented to a health practitioner without delay.

It is a fact that dapoxetine which is in the group of SSRIs can have serious effects on the mood and mental state of a man who takes these pills. Therefore, most importantly, it is necessary to observe the state of the individual's mental health. Mention should be made to the patients to report any alteration in their mental status. Symptoms such as severe neuropsychiatric perturbation might require the provider to modify the dose or even stop the medication.

However, study has shown that dapoxetine , through its usage for the treatment of PE, alters sexual functions in the long run. Therefore, if sexual dysfunction occurs, speaking with the healthcare provider becomes mandatory in order to assess if dapoxetine continued use is possible or whether other treatment options need to be sought.

THE END